I0408207

KETOGENIC DIET
COOKBOOK

45 Ketogenic Recipes for YOUR Healthy Life (breakfast, lunch, dinner)

Stella Parker

© **Copyright 2017 by Stella Parker - All rights reserved.**

This document is geared towards providing exact and reliable information in regards to the topic and issue covered. The publication is sold with the idea that the publisher is not required to render accounting, officially permitted, or otherwise, qualified services. If advice is necessary, legal or professional, a practiced individual in the profession should be ordered.

From a Declaration of Principles which was accepted and approved equally by a Committee of the American Bar Association and a Committee of Publishers and Associations.

In no way is it legal to reproduce, duplicate, or transmit any part of this document in either electronic means or in printed format. Recording of this publication is strictly prohibited and any storage of this document is not allowed unless with written permission from the publisher. All rights reserved.

The information provided herein is stated to be truthful and consistent, in that any liability, in terms of inattention or otherwise, by any usage or abuse of any policies, processes, or directions contained within is the solitary and utter responsibility of the recipient reader. Under no circumstances will any legal responsibility or blame be held against the publisher for any reparation, damages, or monetary loss due to the information herein, either directly or indirectly. Respective authors own all copyrights not held by the publisher.

The information herein is offered for informational purposes solely and is universal as so. The presentation of the information is without contract or any type of guarantee assurance.

The trademarks that are used are without any consent, and the publication of the trademark is without permission or backing by the trademark owner. All trademarks and brands within this book are for clarifying purposes only and are the owned by the owners themselves, not affiliated with this document.

Table of Contents

5

BREAKFAST RECIPES

1-Avocado Bacon Breakfast Burrito

Total Time: 25 minutes

Serves: 2 Servings

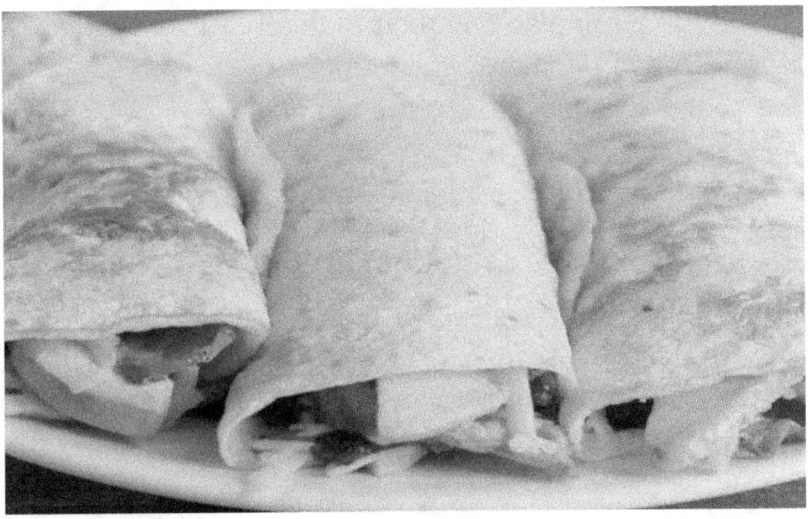

Ingredients:
- 1/2 avocado, sliced
- 2 eggs
- 4 bacon strips, cooked
- 1 medium tomato, sliced
- 1 cup romaine lettuce, chopped
- 2 tbsp mayonnaise
- 2 tsp butter
- Pepper

- Salt

Directions:
1. Whisk eggs with pepper and salt.
2. Melt 1 tsp butter in pan over medium heat.
3. Pour half egg mixture into a hot pan and spread evenly. Cover and cook for a minute.
4. Flip to other side and cook until done.
5. Transfer crepe to dish and spread half mayonnaise on crepe then top with avocado, bacon, tomato, and lettuce.
6. Season with pepper and salt.
7. Roll and serve.
8. Repeat with remaining egg mixture.

Nutritional Value (Amount per Serving):
- Calories 472
- Fat 38.9 g
- Carbohydrates 10.8 g
- Sugar 2.6 g
- Protein 21.2 g
- Cholesterol 219 mg

2-Healthy Breakfast Muffins

Total Time: 25 minutes

Serves: 12 Servings

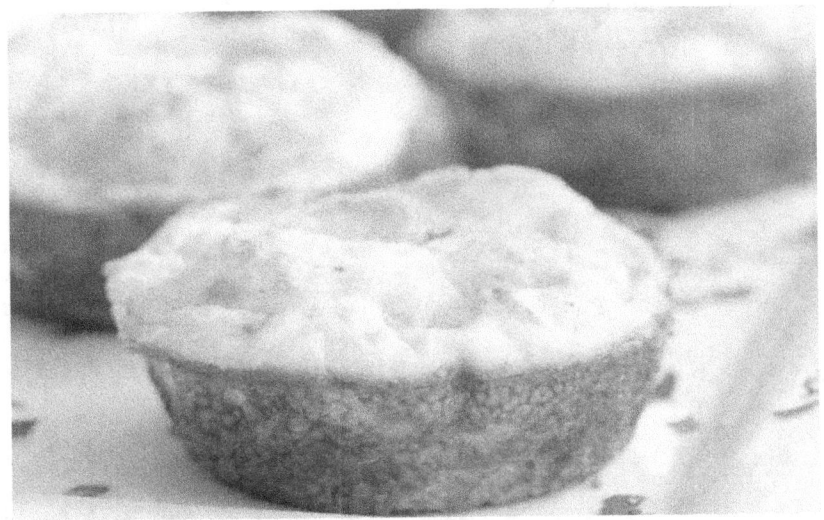

Ingredients:
- 2 scoops whey protein powder
- 4 tbsp butter, melted
- 8 eggs
- 8 oz cream cheese

Directions:
1. Add all ingredients into the large bowl.
2. Using beater, beat until completely combined.
3. Spray muffin pan with cooking spray.
4. Pour batter evenly in prepared muffin pan and bake at 350 F for 25 minutes.

5. Serve and enjoy.

Nutritional Value (Amount per Serving):

- Calories 168
- Fat 14.1 g
- Carbohydrates 1.4 g
- Sugar 0.5 g
- Protein 9.4 g
- Cholesterol 166 mg

3-Easy Coconut Pancakes

Total Time: 20 minutes

Serves: 12 Servings

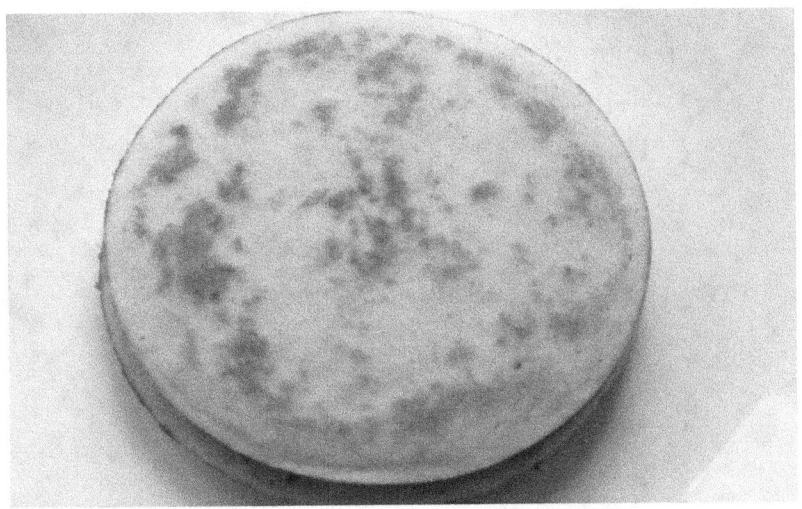

Ingredients:
- 3 eggs
- 1/2 tsp baking powder
- 1/4 cup coconut flour
- 1/2 tsp vanilla
- 1 packet stevia
- 1/4 cup heavy cream
- 1/4 cup butter, melted
- Pinch of salt

Directions:

1. Add eggs, vanilla, salt, stevia, heavy cream, and butter in bowl and whisk well.
2. Combine together baking powder and coconut flour.
3. Add dry ingredients into the wet mixture and mix well.
4. Spray pan with cooking spray and heat over medium heat.
5. Scoop 2 tbsp batter onto hot pan and cook for 4 minutes then flip and cook for another 2 minutes.
6. Serve and enjoy.

Nutritional Value (Amount per Serving):
- Calories 60
- Fat 5.9 g
- Carbohydrates 0.6 g
- Sugar 0.1 g
- Protein 1.5 g
- Cholesterol 55 mg

4-Spinach Cheese Breakfast Casserole

Total Time: 55 minutes

Serves: 8 Servings

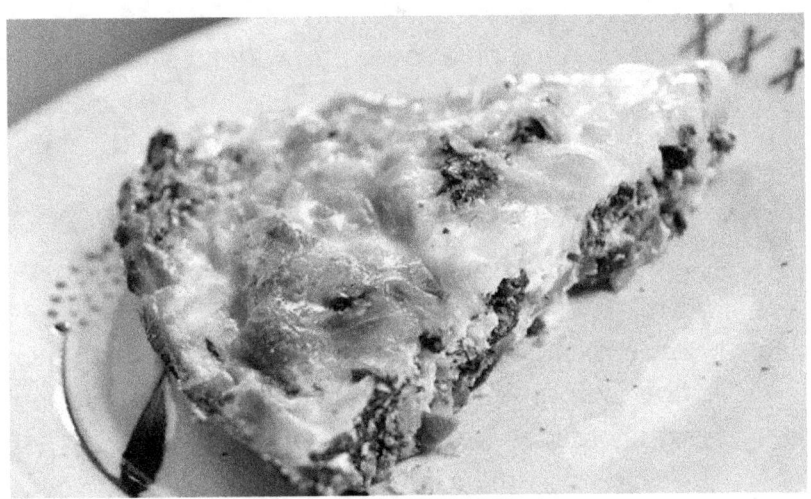

Ingredients:
- 6 eggs, beaten
- 12 oz baby spinach
- 12 oz cheddar cheese, grated
- 16 oz cottage cheese
- 4 tbsp butter, unsalted
- 2 garlic cloves, minced
- 1 medium onion, chopped
- 3 green onion, sliced
- 1/2 lb mushrooms, sliced
- 1/2 tsp pepper
- 1/2 tsp salt

Directions:
1. Preheat the oven to 350 F.
2. Spray baking dish with cooking spray and set aside.
3. Melt butter in pan over medium heat.
4. Add onion, garlic and mushrooms and sauté for 4 minutes or until onion are softened.
5. Add spinach and cover pan with lid and cook for 5 minutes or until spinach wilted.
6. Set aside to cool and drain excess liquid.
7. In a bowl, whisk together eggs, cheddar cheese, cottage cheese, pepper, and salt.
8. Add cooked mushroom and spinach and stir well.
9. Pour mixture into the prepared baking dish and bake in preheated oven for 45 minutes or until lightly golden brown.
10. Serve and enjoy.

Nutritional Value (Amount per Serving):
- Calories 358
- Fat 25.9 g
- Carbohydrates 7.4 g
- Sugar 2.1 g
- Protein 25 g
- Cholesterol 191 mg

5-Baked Eggs in Avocado

Total Time: 20 minutes

Serves: 2 Servings

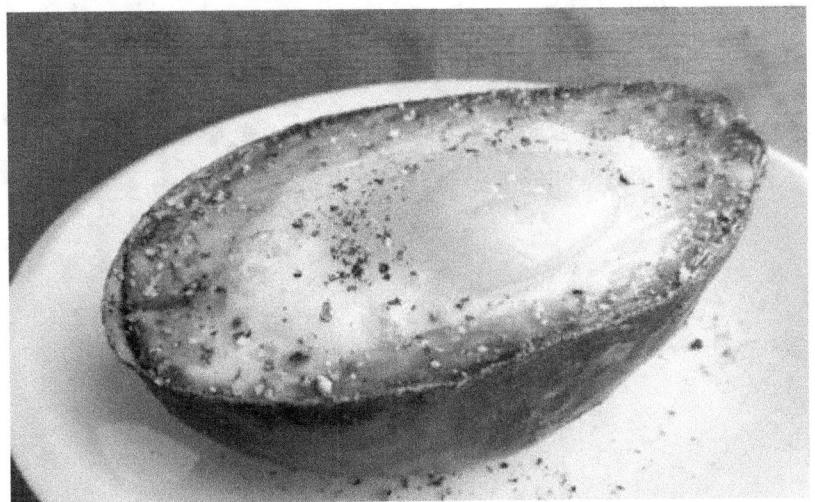

Ingredients:
- 2 large eggs
- 1 medium avocado, cut in half and pitted
- Pepper
- Salt

Directions:
1. Scoop out some avocado flesh to fit eggs in avocado.
2. Break egg into the center of each avocado half.
3. Season with pepper and salt.

4. Bake at 400 F for 15 minutes or until egg whites are set.
5. Serve and enjoy.

Nutritional Value (Amount per Serving):
- Calories 277
- Fat 24.6 g
- Carbohydrates 9.1 g
- Sugar 0.9 g
- Protein 8.2 g
- Cholesterol 186 mg

6-Delicious Coconut Waffles

Total Time: 30 minutes

Serves: 5 Servings

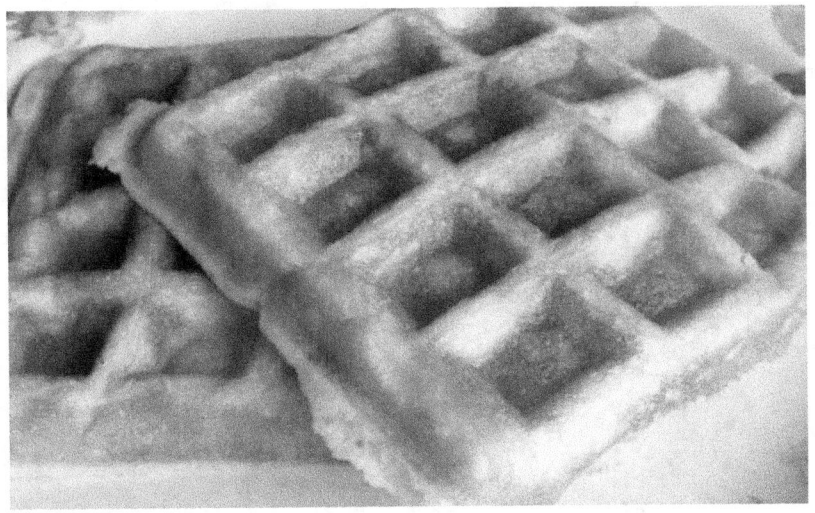

Ingredients:
- 5 eggs, separated
- 4.5 oz butter, melted
- 3 tbsp milk
- 1 tsp vanilla extract
- 1 tsp baking powder
- 3 tbsp granulated sweetener
- 4 tbsp coconut flour

Directions:
1. Add egg whites in bowl and beat until stiff peaks form.

2. Take another bowl and whisk together egg yolks, baking powder, sweetener, and coconut flour.
3. Add slowly butter and whisk until smooth.
4. Add vanilla and milk. Mix well.
5. Add egg whites in egg yolk mixture and fold gently.
6. Heat waffle iron and spray with cooking spray.
7. Pour waffle mixture into the hot waffle iron and cook until golden brown from both the sides.
8. Serve and enjoy.

Nutritional Value (Amount per Serving):
- Calories 302
- Fat 26.9 g
- Carbohydrates 7.8 g
- Sugar 1.7 g
- Protein 7.7 g
- Cholesterol 219 mg

7-Vegetable Egg Scramble

Total Time: 20 minutes

Serves: 1 Serving

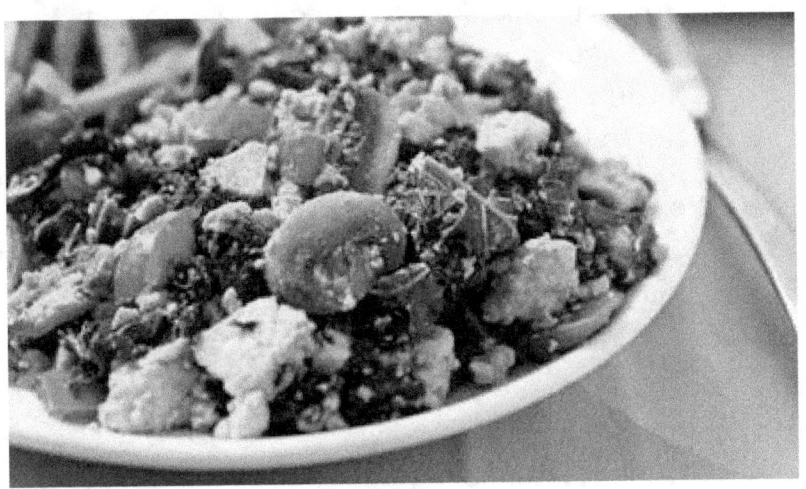

Ingredients:
- 3 eggs, beaten
- 1 tbsp coconut oil
- 2 ham slices, chopped
- 1/2 cup spinach, chopped
- 1/4 cup bell peppers, chopped
- 4 Bella mushrooms, sliced
- Pepper
- Salt

Directions:
1. Melt half tablespoon of coconut oil in pan over medium heat.

2. Add vegetables and ham and sauté for 5 minutes.
3. Heat remaining oil in another pan and add beaten eggs into the pan and cook over medium heat, stir constantly to prevent overcooking.
4. Season cooked eggs with pepper and salt.
5. Add sautéed vegetables and ham in egg mixture and mix well.
6. Serve hot and enjoy.

Nutritional Value (Amount per Serving):
- Calories 414
- Fat 31.7 g
- Carbohydrates 6.6 g
- Sugar 2.8 g
- Protein 27.2 g
- Cholesterol 523 mg

8-Almond Cinnamon Breakfast Porridge

Total Time: 15 minutes

Serves: 2 Servings

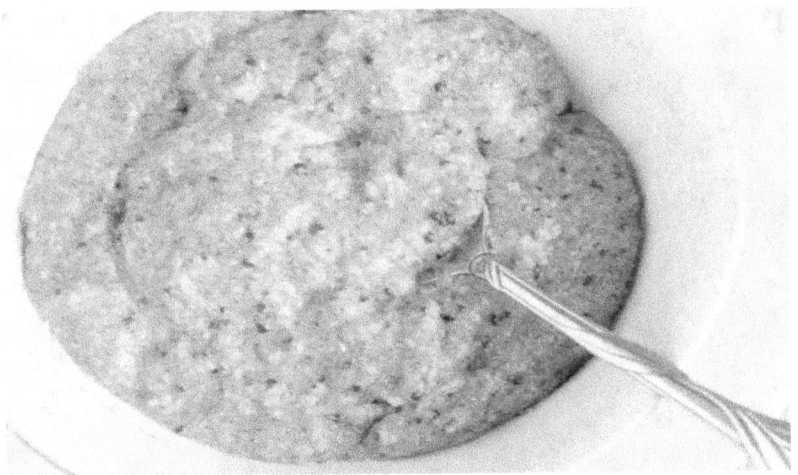

Ingredients:
- 1/2 cup ground almonds
- 1 tsp ground cinnamon
- 1 tsp stevia
- 3/4 cup coconut cream
- Pinch of cloves
- Pinch of nutmeg

Directions:
1. Add coconut cream in saucepan and heat over medium heat until melted.
2. Add stevia and ground almonds and stir well.

3. Stir constantly for 5 minutes over medium heat until thicken.
4. Add spices and stir well.
5. Serve hot and enjoy.

Nutritional Value (Amount per Serving):

- Calories 348
- Fat 33.4 g
- Carbohydrates 11.2 g
- Sugar 4.1 g
- Protein 7.2 g
- Cholesterol 0 mg

9-Chocolate Strawberry Granola

Total Time: 10 minutes

Serves: 1 Serving

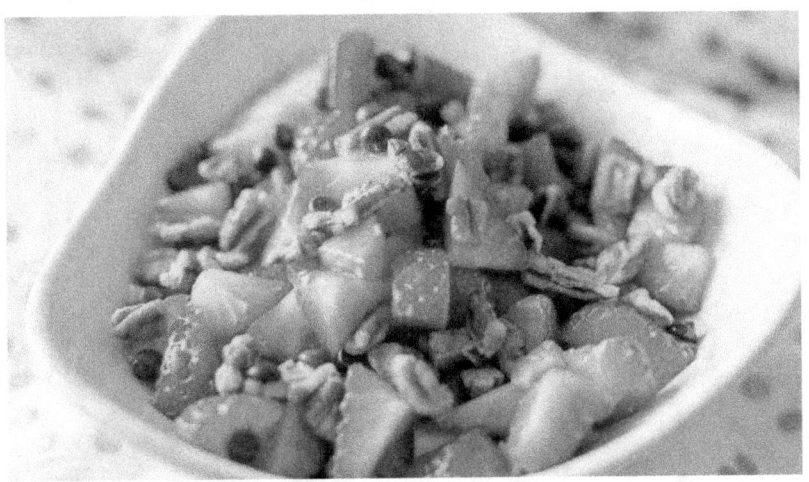

Ingredients:
- 6 fresh strawberries, chopped
- 2 tbsp pecans, chopped
- 2 tbsp chocolate chips
- Fresh lemon juice

Directions:
1. Add all ingredients into the serving bowl and mix well.
2. Serve immediately and enjoy.

Nutritional Value (Amount per Serving):
- Calories 330

- Fat 26.5 g
- Carbohydrates 22 g
- Sugar 15.4 g
- Protein 5.1 g
- Cholesterol 5 mg

10-Quick Cashew Almond Oatmeal

Total Time: 10 minutes

Serves: 1 Serving

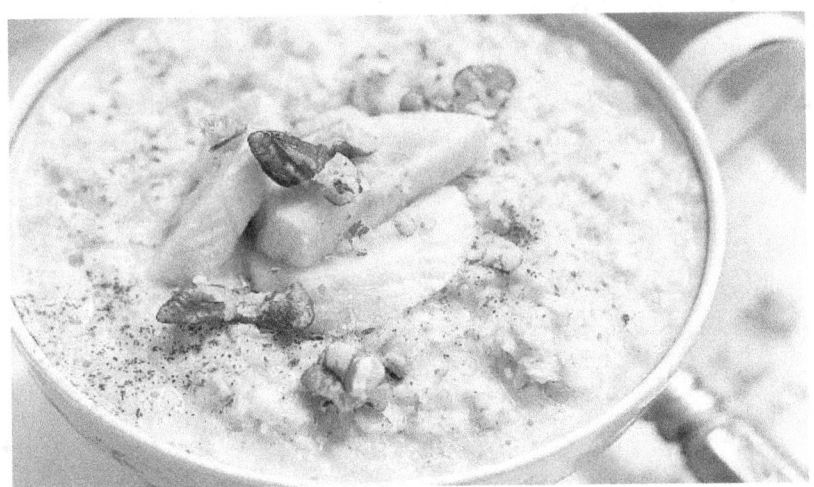

Ingredients:
- 1/2 banana, mashed
- 1/4 tsp cinnamon
- 1/2 cup cashew milk
- 2 tbsp almond flour
- 2 tbsp coconut, shredded and unsweetened
- Pinch of salt

Directions:
1. Add all ingredients into the microwave safe bowl and stir well.
2. Place in microwave and microwave for 2 minutes.

3. Stir well and top with your choice of topping.
4. Serve and enjoy.

Nutritional Value (Amount per Serving):
- Calories 128
- Fat 7.0 g
- Carbohydrates 16.7 g
- Sugar 7.9 g
- Protein 1.8 g
- Cholesterol 0 mg

11-Mix Berry Cereal

Total Time: 10 minutes

Serves: 1 Serving

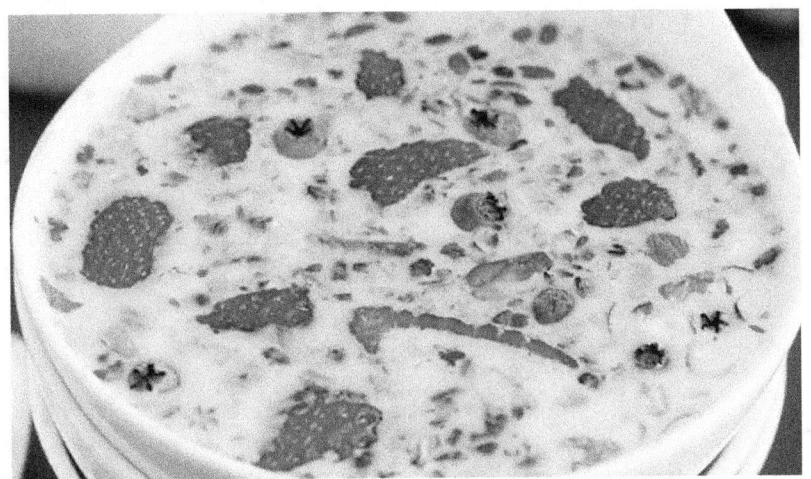

Ingredients:
- 2 tbsp walnuts, chopped
- 3 tbsp pecans, chopped
- 3 tbsp almonds, chopped
- 2 tbsp blueberries
- 2 fresh strawberries, chopped
- 1 tbsp sweetener

Directions:
1. Add all ingredients into the serving bowl and mix well.
2. Add unsweetened almond milk and stir well.
3. Serve and enjoy.

Nutritional Value (Amount per Serving):

- Calories 225
- Fat 19.0 g
- Carbohydrates 12.0 g
- Sugar 3.9 g
- Protein 7.9 g
- Cholesterol 0 mg

12-Cinnamon Sweet Potato Smoothie

Total Time: 5 minutes

Serves: 2 Servings

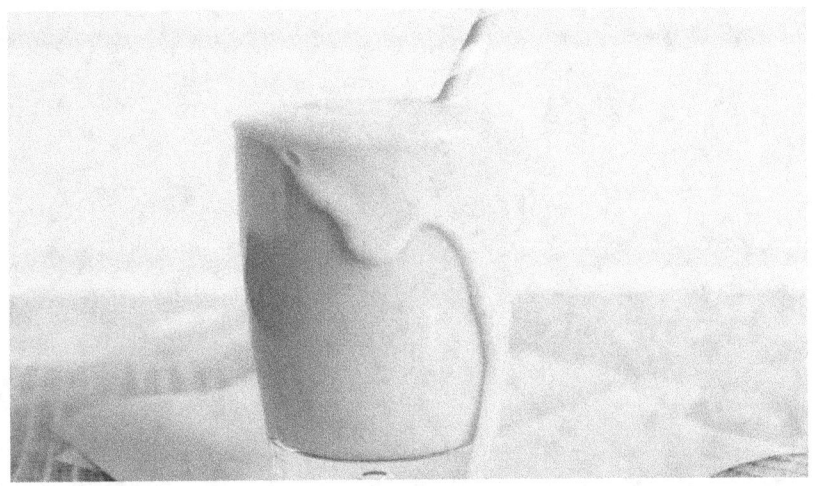

Ingredients:
- 1 small sweet potato, cube
- 1/4 papaya
- 1 medium carrot
- 1 cup almond milk, unsweetened
- 1/2 tsp cinnamon

Directions:
1. Add all ingredients into the blender and blend until smooth.
2. Serve and enjoy.

Nutritional Value (Amount per Serving):

- Calories 334
- Fat 28.8 g
- Carbohydrates 20.6 g
- Sugar 10.5 g
- Protein 3.8 g
- Cholesterol 0 mg

13-Pumpkin Coconut Quinoa Porridge

Total Time: 20 minutes

Serves: 4 Servings

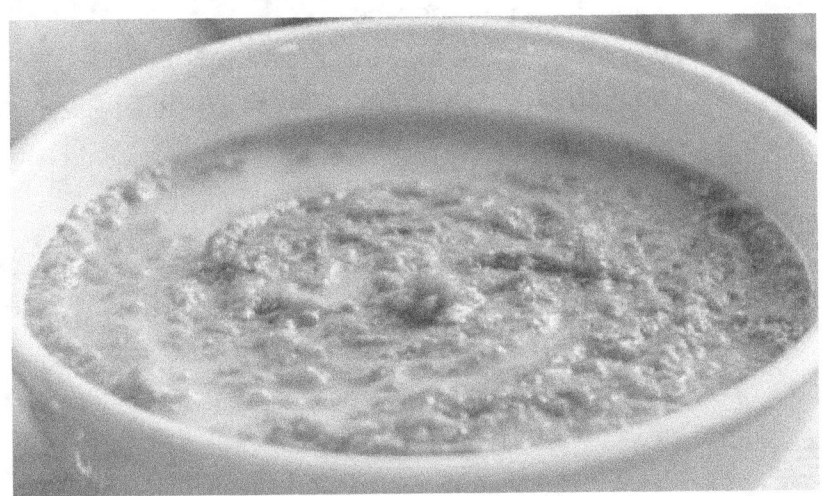

Ingredients:
- 1 cup quinoa, rinsed and drained
- 1/2 cup pumpkin puree
- 2 tbsp maple syrup
- 2 tbsp ground flaxseeds
- 1/8 tsp cloves
- 1/2 tsp ginger
- 1/8 tsp sea salt
- 2 tbsp coconut flakes
- 4 tbsp walnuts, chopped
- 1 tsp cinnamon
- 1 cup almond milk

Directions:
1. In a saucepan add 1 cup almond milk and 1 cup water. Bring to boil over medium heat.
2. Add pumpkin puree, quinoa, ginger, cinnamon, salt and cloves.
3. Reduce heat to low and simmer for 10 minutes or until liquid is absorbed.
4. Turn off the heat and stir in flaxseeds.
5. Top with coconut flakes, maple syrup, and walnuts.
6. Serve and enjoy.

Nutritional Value (Amount per Serving):
- Calories 271
- Fat 9.3 g
- Carbohydrates 39.3 g
- Sugar 7.3 g
- Protein 9.0 g
- Cholesterol 0 mg

14-Vegetable Omelet

Total Time: 20 minutes

Serves: 1 Serving

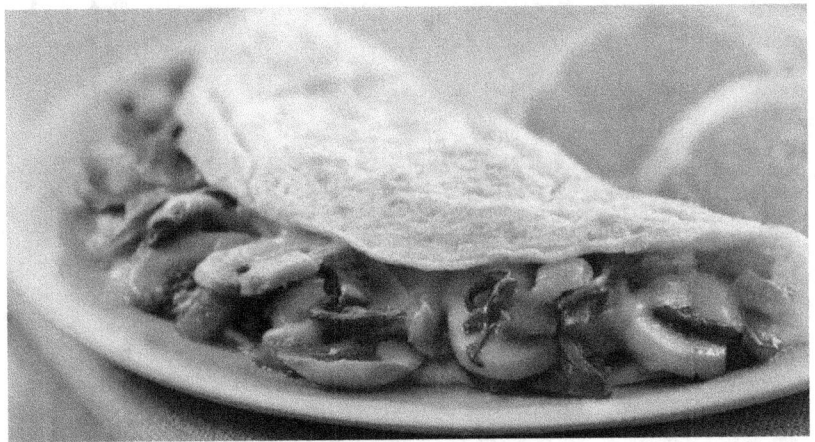

Ingredients:
- 2 eggs
- 4 cherry tomato, halved
- 1 bell pepper, sliced
- 2 button mushroom, sliced
- Pepper
- Salt

Directions:
1. Crack the eggs into the bowl and season with pepper and salt. Whisk well.
2. Spray pan with cooking spray and heat over the medium-high heat.

3. Add tomato, bell pepper, and mushroom, sauté for 4 minutes.
4. Transfer sauté veggies in plate and turn heat to low.
5. Pour egg mixture into the pan and cook for 3 minutes.
6. After 3 minutes flip it over and place sauté veggies on half the omelet and cover the veggies with the other half of the omelet.
7. Serve hot and enjoy.

Nutritional Value (Amount per Serving):

- Calories 171
- Fat 9.2 g
- Carbohydrates 9.1 g
- Sugar 6.3
- Protein 13.4 g
- Cholesterol 327 mg

15-Easy Beef Patties

Total Time: 30 minutes

Serves: 3 Servings

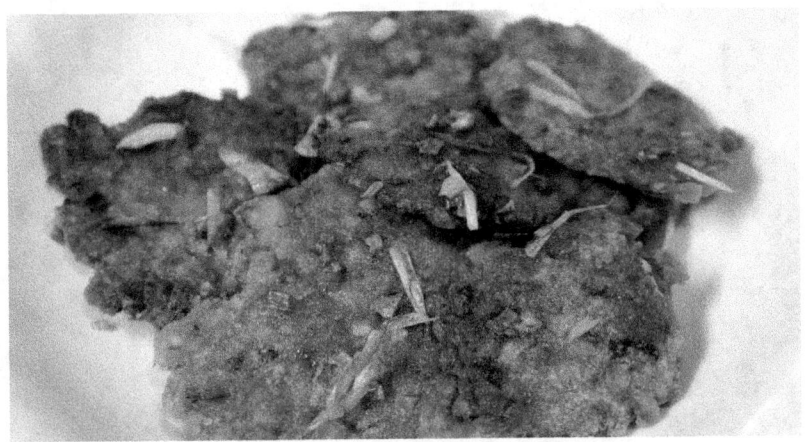

Ingredients:
- 1 lb ground beef
- 1/2 tbsp sage, chopped
- 1/2 tbsp butter
- 1/2 tbsp rosemary, chopped
- 1/2 tbsp thyme, chopped
- 1/2 tsp sea salt

Directions:
1. In a mixing bowl, add ground beef, salt, rosemary, thyme and sage mix well until combined.
2. Make six round shape patties.
3. Melt butter in pan over the medium heat.

4. Place patties in a hot pan and cook for 6 minutes on each side or until lightly browned.
5. Serve and enjoy.

Nutritional Value (Amount per Serving):
- Calories 302
- Fat 11.5 g
- Carbohydrates 0.8 g
- Protein 46.0 g
- Cholesterol 140 mg

LUNCH RECIPES

16-Delicious Grilled Shrimp

Total Time: 40 minutes

Serves: 4 Servings

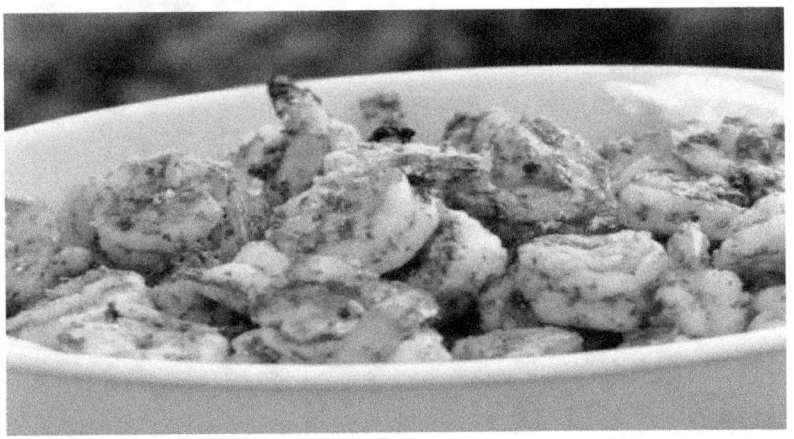

Ingredients:
- 1 lb shrimp, peeled and deveined
- 1 tbsp lemon juice
- 1 tbsp olive oil
- 2 tbsp parmesan cheese, grated
- 1 tbsp pine nuts, toasted
- 1 garlic clove
- 1/2 cup basil
- Pepper
- Salt

Directions:

1. Add basil, lemon juice, cheese, pine nuts, garlic, pepper, and salt in blender and blend until smooth.
2. Add shrimp and basil pest in mixing bowl and mix well.
3. Place shrimp bowl in refrigerator for 20 minutes.
4. Skewer marinated shrimp and grill over medium heat for 3 minutes on each side or until cooked.
5. Serve and enjoy.

Nutritional Value (Amount per Serving):

- Calories 223
- Fat 11.2 g
- Carbohydrates 2.2 g
- Sugar 0.2 g
- Protein 27.2 g
- Cholesterol 241 mg

17-Keto Low Carb Bowl

Total Time: 20 minutes

Serves: 6 Servings

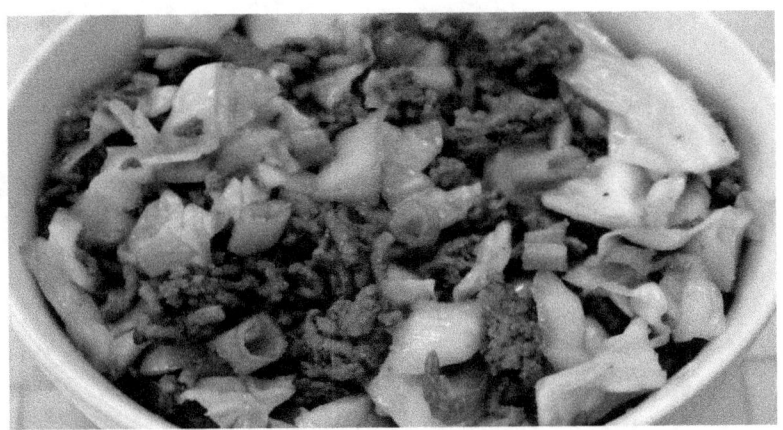

Ingredients:
- 1 lb ground pork
- 2 green onion stalks, chopped
- 2 tbsp chicken broth
- 1 tsp ground ginger
- 1 garlic clove, minced
- 4 tbsp soy sauce
- 1 tbsp sesame oil
- 1/2 onion, sliced
- 1 head of cabbage, sliced
- Pepper
- Salt

Directions:

1. Heat pan over medium heat.
2. Add ground pork in hot pan and cook until lightly brown.
3. Add oil and onion in pan with ground pork and mix well. Cook over medium heat.
4. In small bowl, combine together ginger, garlic, and soy sauce.
5. Pour bowl mixture into the pan and mix well.
6. Add remaining ingredients into the pan, stir well and cook for 3 minutes.
7. Serve warm and enjoy.

Nutritional Value (Amount per Serving):
- Calories 264
- Fat 18.6 g
- Carbohydrates 9.4 g
- Sugar 4.5 g
- Protein 15.5 g
- Cholesterol 54 mg

18-Gluten-free Caesar Salad

Total Time: 20 minutes

Serves: 4 Servings

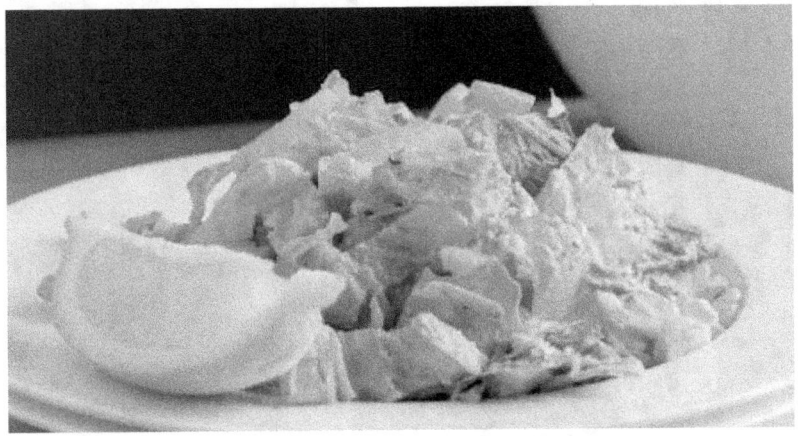

Ingredients:

- 12 cups romaine lettuce, chopped
- 4 tbsp hemp seeds
- 2 tsp Dijon mustard
- 1 tbsp capers
- 1 tbsp caper brine
- 3 garlic cloves, minced
- 2 tbsp water
- 3 tbsp fresh lemon juice
- 1 ripe avocado
- Pepper
- Salt

Directions:

1. Add avocado, pepper, salt, mustard, capers, caper brine, garlic, water, and lemon juice in blender and blend until smooth.
2. Pour avocado mixture and hemp seeds in large mixing bowl and mix well.
3. Add chopped romaine lettuce in bowl and toss well.
4. Serve immediately and enjoy.

Nutritional Value (Amount per Serving):

- Calories 168
- Fat 12.5 g
- Carbohydrates 5.2 g
- Sugar 3.9 g
- Protein 6.6 g
- Cholesterol 0 mg

19-Chicken Garlic Avocado Salad

Total Time: 10 minutes

Serves: 4 Servings

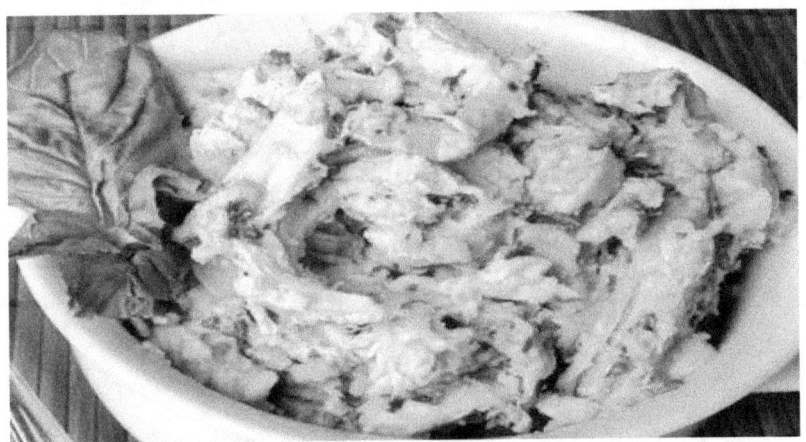

Ingredients:

- 1 cup chicken breasts, cooked and cut into 1/2 inch cubes
- 1 tbsp onion, minced
- 1 tbsp fresh cilantro, minced
- 1/2 tbsp fresh lime juice
- 1 tbsp sour cream
- 1/2 ripe avocado, pitted and peeled
- 1/4 tsp garlic powder
- Pepper
- Salt

Directions:

1. In a bowl, add chicken, avocado, garlic powder, onion, cilantro, lime juice and sour cream. Mix well.
2. Season with pepper and salt.
3. Serve and enjoy.

Nutritional Value (Amount per Serving):
- Calories 127
- Fat 8.1 g
- Carbohydrates 2.8 g
- Sugar 0.3 g
- Protein 10.8 g
- Cholesterol 32 mg

20-Healthy Green Beans with Nuts and Cheese

Total Time: 15 minutes

Serves: 3 Servings

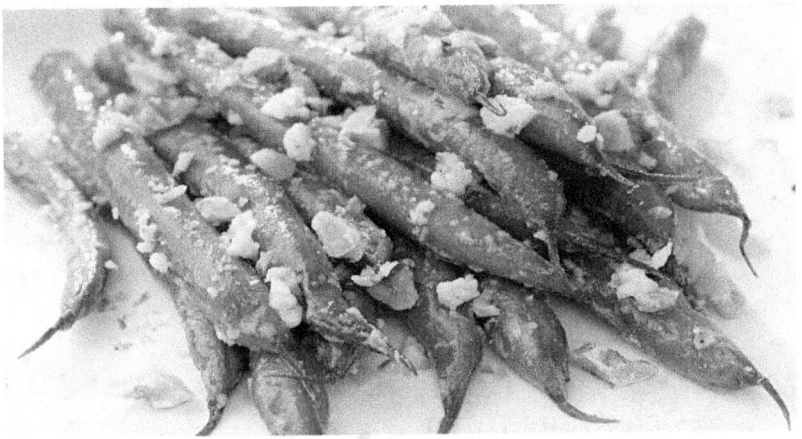

Ingredients:
- 1 lb green beans, trimmed
- 2 tbsp walnuts, chopped
- 1 oz goat cheese, crumbled
- 1/2 tbsp butter
- 1 large shallot, slices
- 1/2 tbsp olive oil
- Pepper
- Salt

Directions:
1. Add salt and water in large pot and bring to boil.

2. Add green beans in hot water and cook for 2 minutes.
3. Drain beans and set aside.
4. Heat oil in pan over medium heat.
5. Add shallots and cook until soften.
6. Add butter, once butter is melted then add green beans and cook for 3 minutes.
7. Transfer green beans in mixing bowl and toss with cheese, walnuts, pepper and salt.
8. Serve immediately and enjoy.

Nutritional Value (Amount per Serving):
- Calories 171
- Fat 10.9 g
- Carbohydrates 14.3 g
- Sugar 2.4 g
- Protein 7.3 g
- Cholesterol 15 mg

21-Simple Broccoli Stir Fry

Total Time: 20 minutes

Serves: 2 Servings

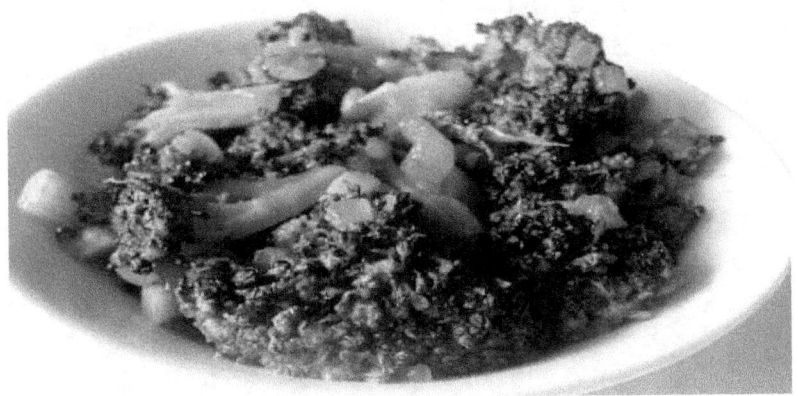

Ingredients:
- 2 cups broccoli florets
- 1/2 tsp apple cider vinegar
- 1/2 tsp garlic, minced
- 1/2 tbsp olive oil
- 1/2 red chili, chopped
- 1/2 tsp honey
- 1/2 onion, sliced

Directions:
1. Boil broccoli florets until tender then drained and set aside.
2. Heat oil in pan over medium heat.

3. Add onion and sauté until soften then add broccoli and toss well.
4. Add remaining ingredients. Stir well and cook for 4 minutes.
5. Serve and enjoy.

Nutritional Value (Amount per Serving):
- Calories 79
- Fat 3.8 g
- Carbohydrates 10.3 g
- Sugar 4.2 g
- Protein 2.9 g
- Cholesterol 0 mg

22-Creamy Egg Salad

Total Time: 20 minutes

Serves: 2 Servings

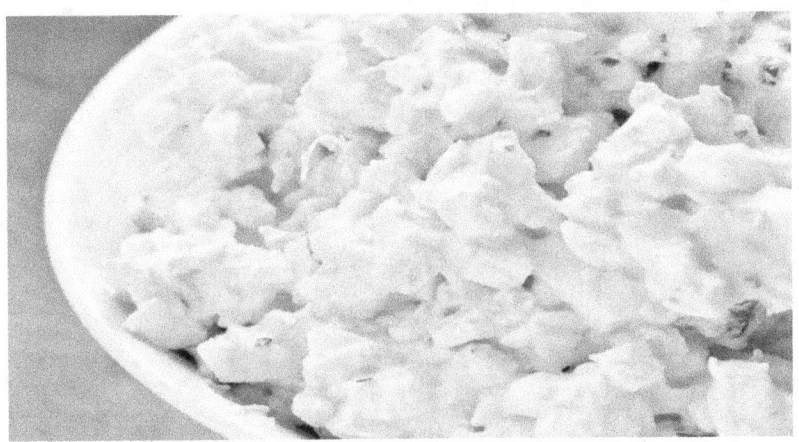

Ingredients:
- 6 eggs, hard boiled, peeled and chopped
- 1 tbsp brown mustard
- 2 celery ribs, diced
- 1/2 bell pepper, diced
- 5 tbsp light mayonnaise
- 2 tbsp fresh parsley, minced
- 4 scallions, sliced
- Pepper
- Salt

Directions:
1. Add all ingredients into the mixing bowl and mix well.

2. Season with pepper and salt.
3. Serve immediately and enjoy.

Nutritional Value (Amount per Serving):
- Calories 363
- Fat 25.6 g
- Carbohydrates 15.7 g
- Sugar 6.1 g
- Protein 18.2 g
- Cholesterol 501 mg

23-Spicy Chicken Lime Cilantro Salad

Total Time: 25 minutes

Serves: 3 Servings

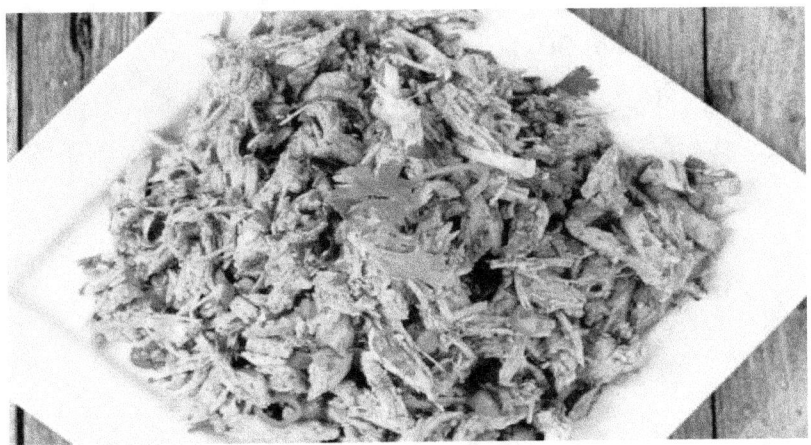

Ingredients:
- 1 1/2 cups chicken, cooked and shredded
- 1/2 fresh lime juice
- 2 tbsp fresh cilantro, chopped
- 1 tsp chili powder
- 1/8 tsp garlic powder
- 1/4 tsp cumin powder
- 1 green onion, sliced
- Pepper
- Salt

Directions:
1. Add all ingredients into the mixing bowl and mix well until combined.

2. Serve immediately and enjoy.

Nutritional Value (Amount per Serving):
- Calories 112
- Fat 2.3 g
- Carbohydrates 1.2 g
- Sugar 0.2 g
- Protein 20.6 g
- Cholesterol 54 mg

24-Coconut Tilapia Fillet

Total Time: 20 minutes

Serves: 4 Servings

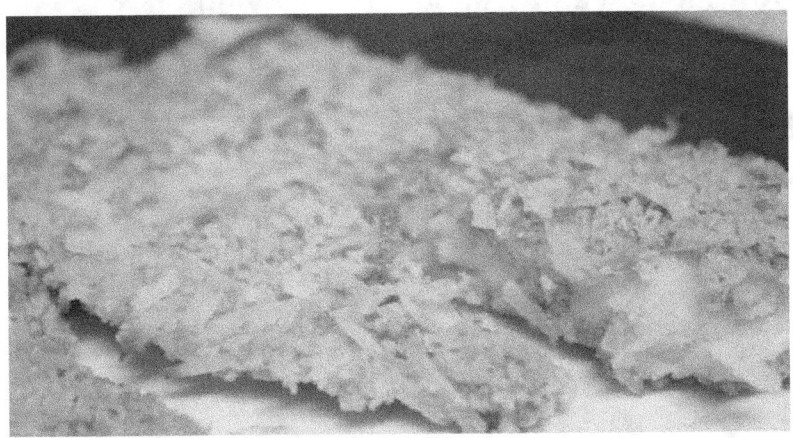

Ingredients:
- 4 tilapia fillets
- 1/2 cup coconut, shredded and unsweetened
- 4 tbsp coconut flour
- 4 tbsp coconut milk
- 3 tbsp olive oil
- Pepper
- Salt

Directions:
1. Heat oil in pan over medium heat.
2. In a dish combine together shredded coconut and coconut flour.

3. Dip tilapia fish in the coconut milk then coat with coconut mixture.
4. Season with pepper and salt,
5. Fry coated fish until golden browned.
6. Serve hot and enjoy.

Nutritional Value (Amount per Serving):
- Calories 330
- Fat 21.9 g
- Carbohydrates 10.4 g
- Sugar 2.1 g
- Protein 24.7 g
- Cholesterol 50 mg

25-Refreshing Cucumber Salad

Total Time: 15 minutes

Serves: 4 Servings

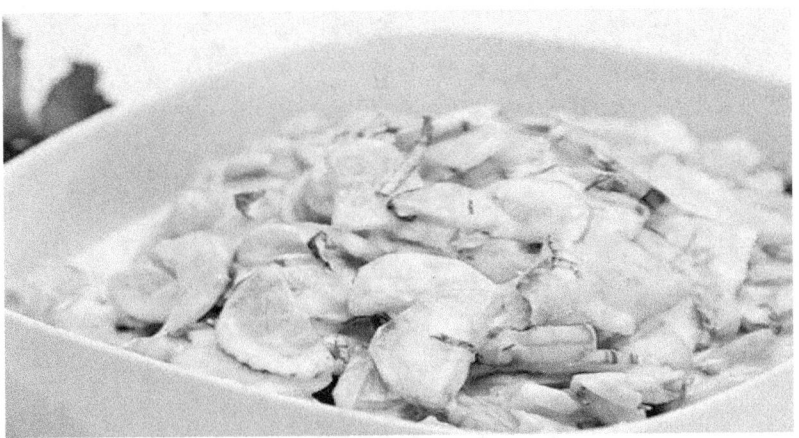

Ingredients:
- 2 medium cucumbers, peeled and sliced
- 1 tbsp white vinegar
- 1 medium onion, sliced
- 1/2 bell pepper, chopped
- 2 tsp fresh dill, chopped
- 1/4 cup sour cream
- 1 tbsp honey
- 1/8 tsp pepper
- 3/4 tsp salt

Directions:
1. In a bowl, add onion, bell pepper, and cucumber. Toss well.

2. In a small bowl, combine together all remaining ingredients and pour over salad.
3. Cover and place in refrigerator.
4. Serve chilled and enjoy.

Nutritional Value (Amount per Serving):
- Calories 87
- Fat 3.3 g
- Carbohydrates 14.5 g
- Sugar 8.8 g
- Protein 2 g
- Cholesterol 6 mg

26-Crunchy Bacon Broccoli Salad

Total Time: 20 minutes

Serves: 8 Servings

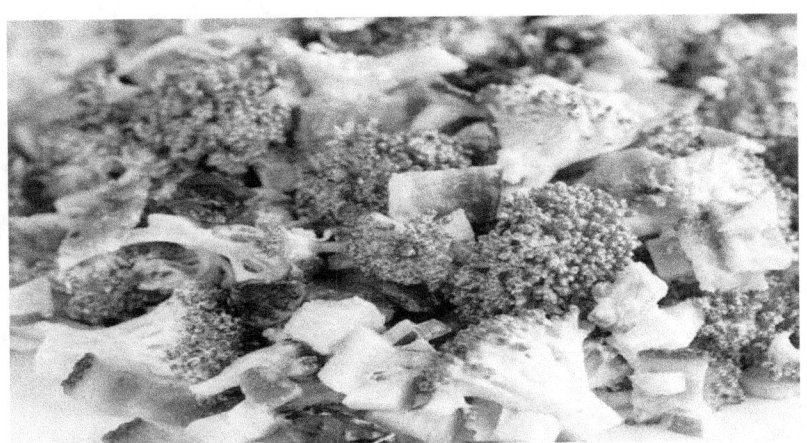

Ingredients:
- 1 lb broccoli, cut into florets
- 4 tbsp cranberries, dried
- 1 tsp olive oil
- 2 tbsp swerve
- 2 tbsp vinegar
- 1 cup mayonnaise
- 1/2 bunch green onion, sliced
- 1/4 lb bacon, cooked and crumble

Directions:
1. Add all ingredients into the large mixing bowl and toss well to combine.
2. Serve and enjoy.

Nutritional Value (Amount per Serving):

- Calories 219
- Fat 16.5 g
- Carbohydrates 18.9 g
- Sugar 10.5 g
- Protein 7.1 g
- Cholesterol 23 mg

27-Yummy Chicken Meatballs

Total Time: 20 minutes

Serves: 9 Servings

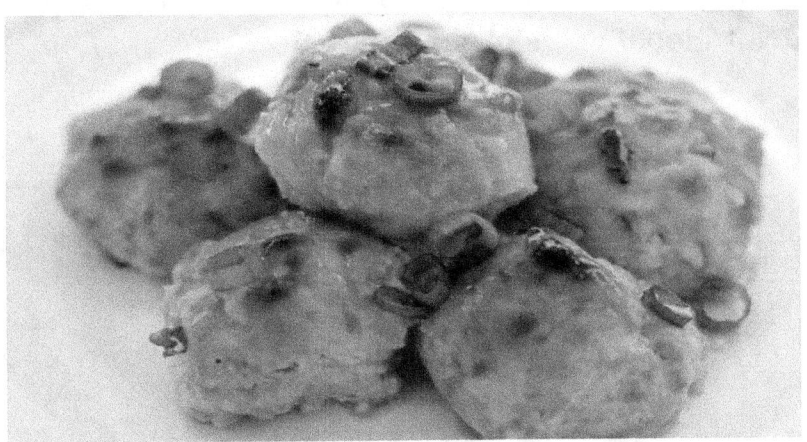

Ingredients:
- 1 egg
- 1 lb ground chicken
- 1/4 cup hot sauce
- 1 tbsp ranch seasoning
- 2 tbsp prepared ranch dressing
- 1/4 cup cheddar cheese
- 1/2 cup almond flour

Directions:
1. Preheat the oven to 500 F.
2. Spray baking tray with cooking spray and set aside.

3. Add all ingredients into the mixing bowl and mix well until combined.
4. Make nine round shape meatballs from mixture and place on prepared baking dish.
5. Bake in preheated oven for 15 minutes.
6. Serve hot and enjoy.

Nutritional Value (Amount per Serving):
- Calories 156
- Fat 11 g
- Carbohydrates 2 g
- Sugar 0 g
- Protein 12 g
- Cholesterol 64 mg

28-Tasty Cauliflower Carrot Peas Fried Rice

Total Time: 30 minutes

Serves: 4 Servings

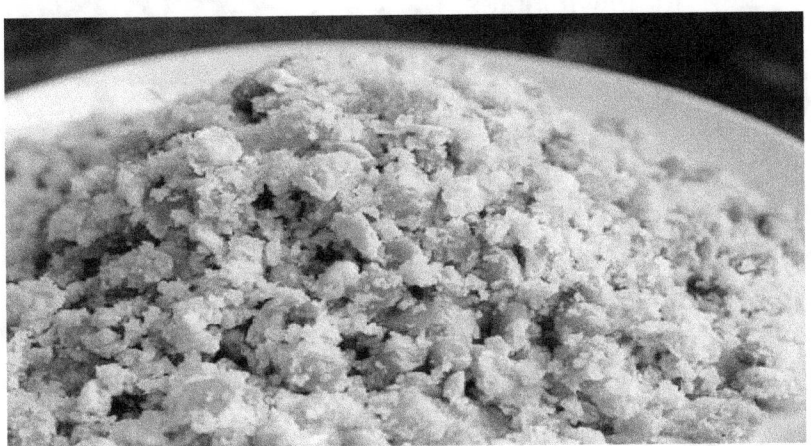

Ingredients:
- 1 large cauliflower head
- 2 tbsp soy sauce
- 2 tbsp olive oil
- 1/2 cup frozen corn, thawed
- 1/2 cup frozen carrots and peas
- 1/2 shallots, minced
- 1 garlic clove, minced

Directions:
1. Preheat the oven to 375 F.
2. Cut cauliflower into the florets.

3. Add cauliflower florets into the food processor and process until it looks like rice.
4. In a large bowl, add cauliflower rice, shallots, garlic, and olive oil.
5. Spread cauliflower mixture on baking tray and roast in preheated oven for 8 minutes.
6. Add veggies in cauliflower mixture and roast for few minutes.
7. Add soy sauce and stir well.
8. Serve warm and enjoy.

Nutritional Value (Amount per Serving):
- Calories 140
- Fat 7.3 g
- Carbohydrates 16.8 g
- Sugar 6 g
- Protein 5.6 g
- Cholesterol 0 mg

29-Delicious Chicken Fajita

Total Time: 40 minutes

Serves: 4 Servings

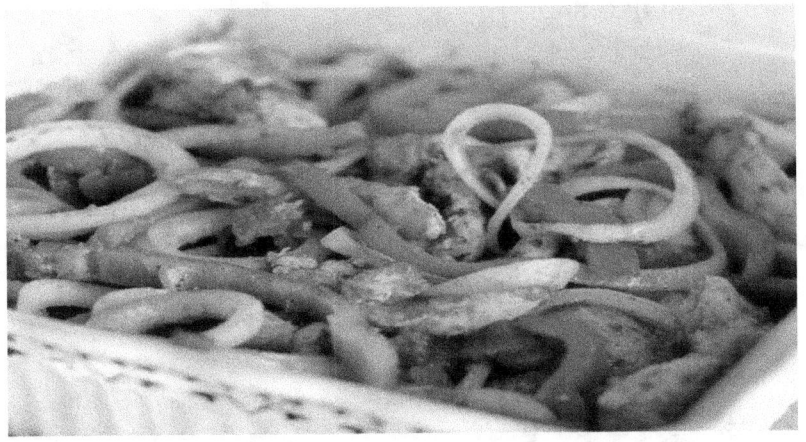

Ingredients:

- 1 lb chicken breasts, skinless and boneless, cut into strips
- 1/2 tsp chili powder
- 2 tsp garlic powder
- 1 tsp onion powder
- 1 tbsp cumin
- 1 ripe tomato, cubed
- 1 bell pepper, sliced
- 1 onion, sliced
- 1 tsp pepper
- 1/4 tsp salt

Directions:

1. Preheat the oven to 190 C/ 375 F.
2. Spray baking dish with cooking spray and set aside.
3. In a mixing bowl, combine together all seasoning ingredients.
4. Add chicken in mixing bowl and mix well with seasoning.
5. Place season chicken on prepare baking dish.
6. Top chicken with vegetables.
7. Bake in preheated oven for 35 minutes.
8. Serve and enjoy.

Nutritional Value (Amount per Serving):
- Calories 254
- Fat 9 g
- Carbohydrates 8.1 g
- Sugar 3.7 g
- Protein 34.2 g
- Cholesterol 101 mg

30-Healthy Broccoli Omelet

Total Time: 20 minutes

Serves: 2 Servings

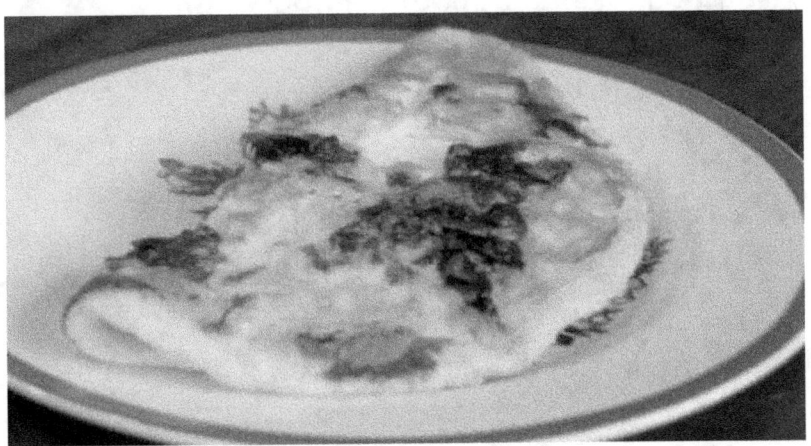

Ingredients:

- 4 eggs
- 1 cup broccoli, chopped and cooked
- 1 tbsp olive oil
- 1 tbsp parsley, chopped
- 1/4 tsp marjoram, dried
- 1/4 tsp pepper
- 1/2 tsp salt

Directions:

1. In a bowl, beat eggs with pepper, marjoram, and salt.
2. Heat olive oil in pan over medium heat.

3. Pour broccoli and eggs mixture in a hot pan and cook until set then flip omelet and cook until lightly golden brown.
4. Garnish with chopped parsley.
5. Serve hot and enjoy.

Nutritional Value (Amount per Serving):
- Calories 203
- Fat 15.9 g
- Carbohydrates 4 g
- Sugar 1.5 g
- Protein 12.4 g
- Cholesterol 327 mg

DINNER RECIPES

31-Tomato Pepper Soup

Total Time: 30 minutes

Serves: 4 Servings

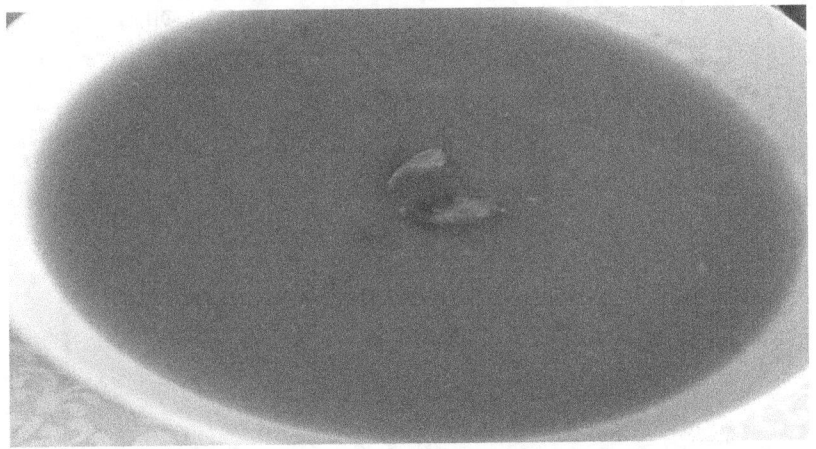

Ingredients:
- 3 cups tomatoes, peeled, seeded and chopped
- 1/2 tsp thyme, chopped
- 4 cups chicken broth, low-sodium
- 1 tbsp garlic, minced
- 1 cup red bell pepper, chopped
- 1 cup onion, chopped
- 1 tsp oregano, chopped
- 1 tbsp basil, chopped
- 2 tbsp tomato paste

- 1 tbsp olive oil
- 1/4 tsp pepper

Directions:

1. Heat oil in saucepan over medium heat.
2. Add garlic, onion, bell pepper, and tomatoes and sauté for 10 minutes.
3. Add all remaining ingredients and stir well to combine.
4. Increase heat to high and bring to boil.
5. Reduce heat to low and cover and simmer for 10 minutes.
6. Remove from heat and using blender, puree the soup until smooth.
7. Serve and enjoy.

Nutritional Value (Amount per Serving):

- Calories 125
- Fat 5.4 g
- Carbohydrates 13.7 g
- Sugar 8 g
- Protein 7.2 g
- Cholesterol 0 mg

32-Roasted Salmon

Total Time: 25 minutes

Serves: 4 Servings

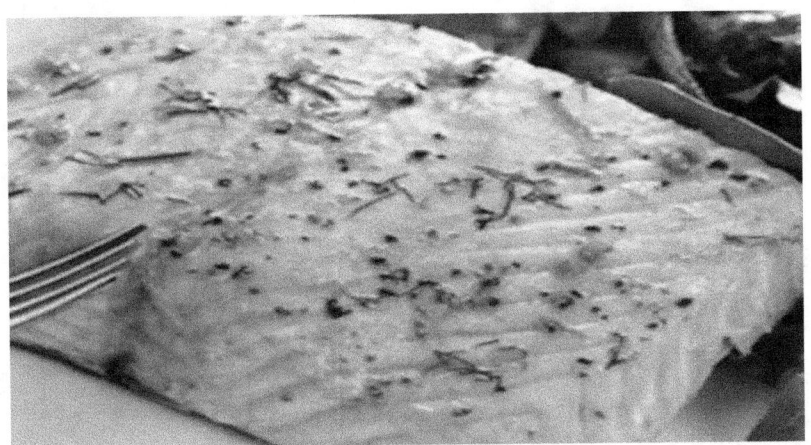

Ingredients:
- 1 lb salmon, slice into fillets
- 1 lemon juice
- 2 tbsp dill, chopped
- 2 tbsp prepared mustard

Directions:
1. Preheat the oven to 450 F.
2. Place salmon fillets in baking tray.
3. Add all remaining ingredients into the bowl and brush over the salmon fillets.
4. Bake in preheated oven for 15 minutes.
5. Serve and enjoy.

Nutritional Value (Amount per Serving):

- Calories 162
- Fat 7.5 g
- Carbohydrates 1.5 g
- Sugar 0.3 g
- Protein 22.7 g
- Cholesterol 50 mg

33-Creamy Pumpkin Tomato Soup

Total Time: 25 minutes

Serves: 4 Servings

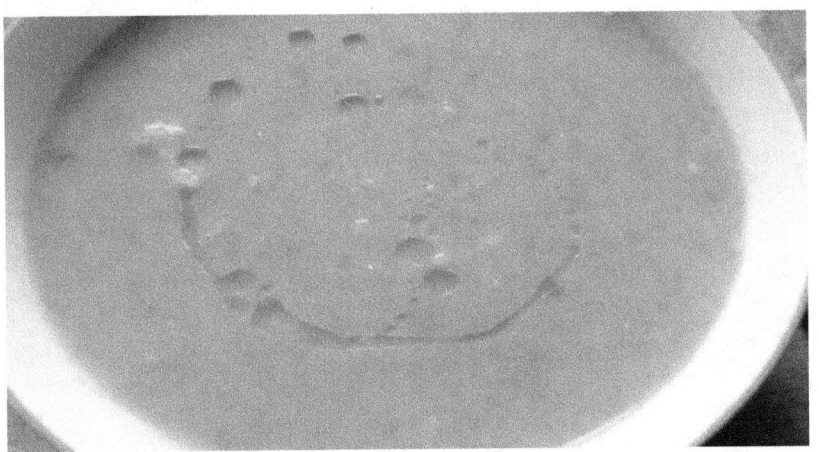

Ingredients:
- 2 cups pumpkin
- 1/2 cup tomato, chopped
- 2 cups vegetable broth, low-sodium
- 1 tsp olive oil
- 1/2 tsp garlic, minced
- 1 1/2 tsp curry powder
- 1/2 tsp paprika
- 1/2 cup onion, chopped

Directions:
1. In a saucepan, add oil, garlic, and onion and sauté for 3 minutes.

2. Add remaining ingredients to the saucepan and bring to boil.
3. Reduce heat and cover and simmer for 10 minutes or until pumpkin is tender.
4. Using blender, puree the soup until smooth and creamy.
5. Serve and enjoy.

Nutritional Value (Amount per Serving):
- Calories 84
- Fat 2.4 g
- Carbohydrates 13.3 g
- Sugar 5.6 g
- Protein 4.3 g
- Cholesterol 0 mg

34-Veggie Tofu Scramble

Total Time: 20 minutes

Serves: 4 Servings

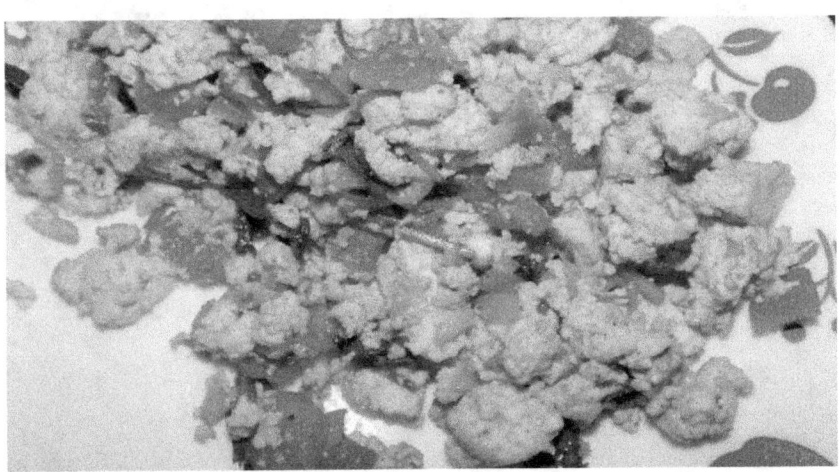

Ingredients:
- 1 lb firm tofu, drained
- 1 cup mushrooms, sliced
- 1 garlic clove, minced
- 1/2 tsp turmeric
- 1 bell pepper, diced
- 1 tomato, diced
- 1 small onion, diced
- 1/2 tsp pepper
- 1/2 tsp salt

Directions:
1. Heat pan over medium heat.

2. Add garlic, onion, tomato, mushrooms, and bell pepper and sauté for 5 minutes.
3. Crumble tofu and add in pan over the vegetables.
4. Add turmeric, pepper, and salt stir well to combine.
5. Cook tofu scramble for another 5 minutes.
6. Serve hot and enjoy.

Nutritional Value (Amount per Serving):

- Calories 105
- Fat 5 g
- Carbohydrates 7.6 g
- Sugar 3.7 g
- Protein 10.6 g
- Cholesterol 0 mg

35-Creamy Asparagus Lemon Thyme Soup

Total Time: 35 minutes

Serves: 4 Servings

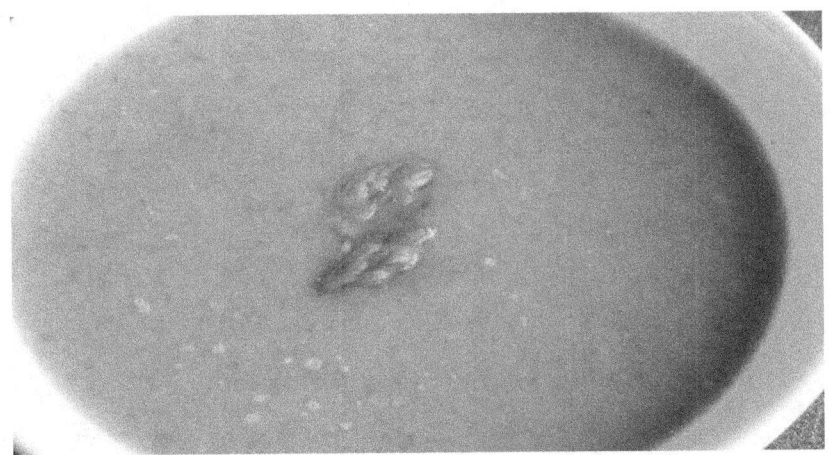

Ingredients:
- 1 lb asparagus, sliced
- 3/4 tsp fresh thyme, chopped
- 1/2 tbsp fresh lemon juice
- 1/4 tsp lemon zest, grated
- 2 cups soy milk
- 2 cups vegetable broth
- 2 tbsp whole wheat flour
- 2 garlic cloves, crushed
- 1 bay leaf
- 1 tsp salt
- Pepper

Directions:

1. In a saucepan add asparagus, garlic, bay leaf, thyme and vegetable broth.
2. Bring to boil over medium high heat for 10 minutes.
3. Remove bay leaf and using blender, puree the soup until smooth.
4. Add flour in saucepan over medium heat then add slowly soy milk and whisk until combined.
5. Now add asparagus mixture, stir well and bring to boil for 5 minutes.
6. Remove from heat and strain.
7. Add lemon juice, lemon zest, salt and pepper.
8. Serve and enjoy.

Nutritional Value (Amount per Serving):

- Calories 126
- Fat 3.1 g
- Carbohydrates 16.4 g
- Sugar 7.5 g
- Protein 9.5 g
- Cholesterol 0 mg

36-Tangy Chicken Roast

Total Time: 45 minutes

Serves: 4 Servings

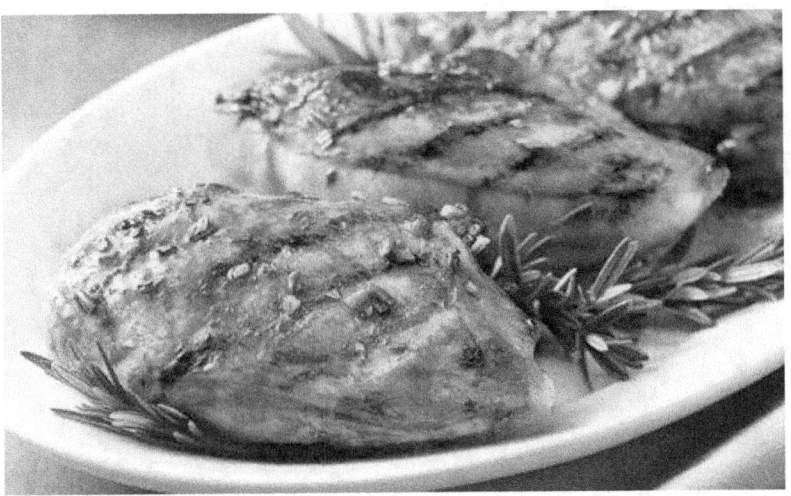

Ingredients:
- 16 oz chicken breasts, skinless
- 1/4 cup orange juice
- 1 garlic clove, chopped
- 1/2 tsp olive oil
- 1 tsp rosemary, chopped
- Pepper

Directions:
1. Preheat the oven to 450 F.
2. Spray baking tray with cooking spray and set aside.
3. Rub garlic and olive oil over the chicken.

4. Season chicken with rosemary and pepper.
5. Place seasoned chicken in prepared baking tray.
6. Pour orange juice over the chicken and bake in preheated oven for 25 minutes.
7. Flip chicken to other side and bake for another 10 minutes.
8. Serve and enjoy.

Nutritional Value (Amount per Serving):
- Calories 230
- Fat 9.1 g
- Carbohydrates 2.1 g
- Sugar 1.3 g
- Protein 33 g
- Cholesterol 101 mg

37-Pepper Mustard Corn Apple Salad

Total Time: 15 minutes

Serves: 4 Servings

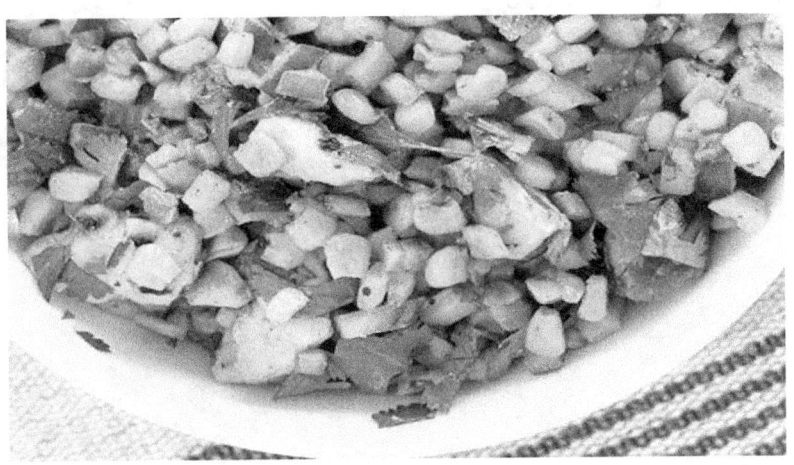

Ingredients:
- 1 tbsp apple cider vinegar
- 1 tsp Dijon mustard
- 1 avocado, peeled and cubed
- 3 tbsp olive oil
- 2 cups corn, cooked
- 1 cup apple, chopped
- 1 cup green bell pepper, diced

Directions:
1. Add corn, apple, avocado, and bell pepper in large bowl.

2. In small bowl, combine together oil, vinegar, and mustard and pour over salad and toss well.
3. Serve immediately and enjoy.

Nutritional Value (Amount per Serving):
- Calories 299
- Fat 21.4 g
- Carbohydrates 28.9 g
- Sugar 10.1 g
- Protein 4 g
- Cholesterol 0 mg

38-Simple Chicken Patties

Total Time: 20 minutes

Serves: 6 Servings

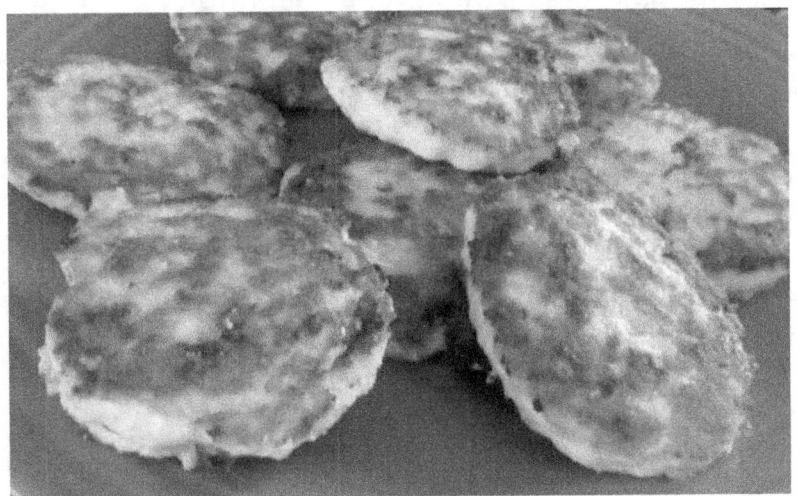

Ingredients:
- 2 cups chicken, cooked and shredded
- 4 green onions, chopped
- 1/2 cup crackers, crushed
- 1/3 cup mayonnaise
- 2 tbsp olive oil
- 2 tbsp lemon juice
- Pepper

Directions:
1. Add all ingredients into the bowl and mix well until combine.

2. Form mixture into six round shape patties.
3. Heat oil in pan over medium heat.
4. Once oil is hot place patties and cook for 3 minutes on each side or until lightly brown.
5. Serve and enjoy.

Nutritional Value (Amount per Serving):
- Calories 192
- Fat 11.8 g
- Carbohydrates 7.1 g
- Sugar 1.3 g
- Protein 14.2 g
- Cholesterol 39 mg

39-Creamy Cauliflower Mash

Total Time: 25 minutes

Serves: 6 Servings

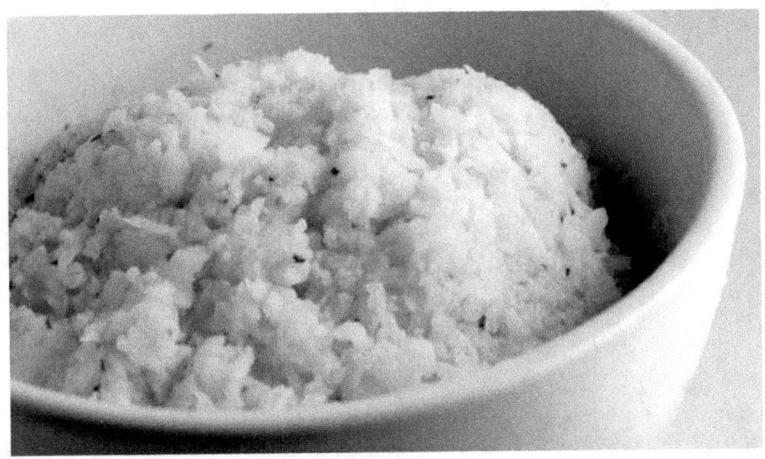

Ingredients:
- 2 cauliflower heads, cut into florets
- 1/2 tsp garlic powder
- 4 tbsp margarine
- 2 tbsp milk
- 1/2 tsp onion powder
- 1/2 tsp black pepper
- 1/2 tsp salt

Directions:
1. Add cauliflower in saucepan and add enough water to cover cauliflower.

2. Cover saucepan with lid and cook over medium heat for 15 minutes.
3. Drain cauliflower well and place in mixing bowl.
4. Add remaining ingredients in bowl and using blender blend until smooth.
5. Serve warm and enjoy.

Nutritional Value (Amount per Serving):
- Calories 94
- Fat 7.8 g
- Carbohydrates 5.5 g
- Sugar 2.5 g
- Protein 2.1 g
- Cholesterol 0 mg

40-Crispy Roasted Cauliflower

Total Time: 40 minutes

Serves: 4 Servings

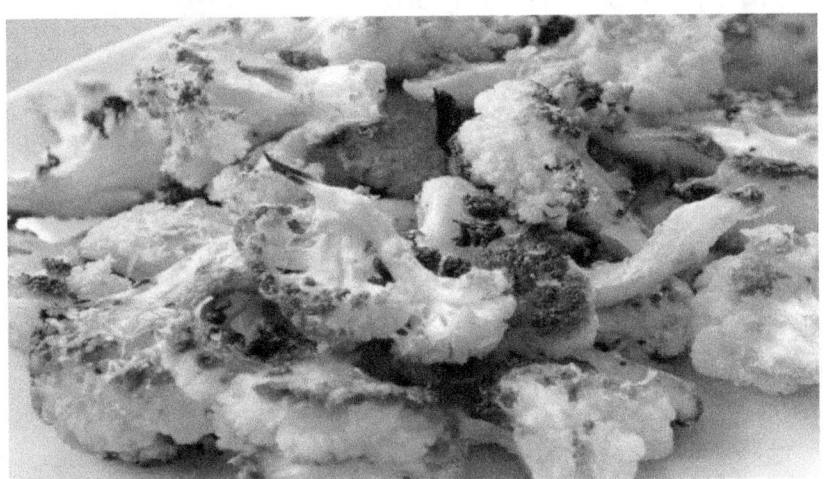

Ingredients:
- 1 cauliflower head, cut into florets
- 1 tbsp olive oil
- 2 tbsp fresh sage, chopped
- 1 garlic clove, minced

Directions:
1. Preheat the oven to 400 F.
2. Spray baking tray with cooking spray.
3. Spread cauliflower florets evenly on prepared baking tray.
4. Bake cauliflower in preheated oven for 30 minutes.

5. Meanwhile, sauté garlic in pan with 1 tbsp oil. Remove from heat and set aside.
6. Add cauliflower, garlic oil and sage in bowl and toss well.
7. Serve and enjoy.

Nutritional Value (Amount per Serving):
- Calories 51
- Fat 3.7 g
- Carbohydrates 4.4 g
- Sugar 1.6 g
- Protein 1.5 g
- Cholesterol 0 mg

41-Roasted Green Beans

Total Time: 35 minutes

Serves: 4 Servings

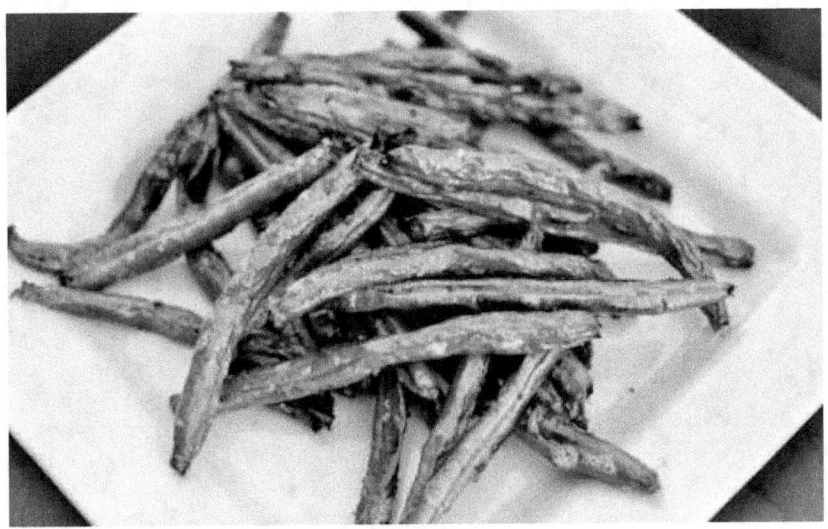

Ingredients:
- 1 lb frozen green beans
- 2 tbsp olive oil
- 1/2 tsp garlic powder
- 1/2 tsp onion powder
- 1/2 tsp pepper
- 1/2 tsp salt

Directions:
1. Spray baking dish with cooking spray and set aside.
2. Preheat the oven to 218 C/ 425 F.

3. In a bowl, add all ingredients and mix well.
4. Spread green beans evenly on prepared baking dish.
5. Bake in oven for 30 minutes.
6. Serve hot and enjoy.

Nutritional Value (Amount per Serving):
- Calories 98
- Fat 7.2 g
- Carbohydrates 8.8 g
- Sugar 1.8 g
- Protein 2.2 g
- Cholesterol 0 mg

42-Lemon Chicken Apple Salad

Total Time: 25 minutes

Serves: 1 Serving

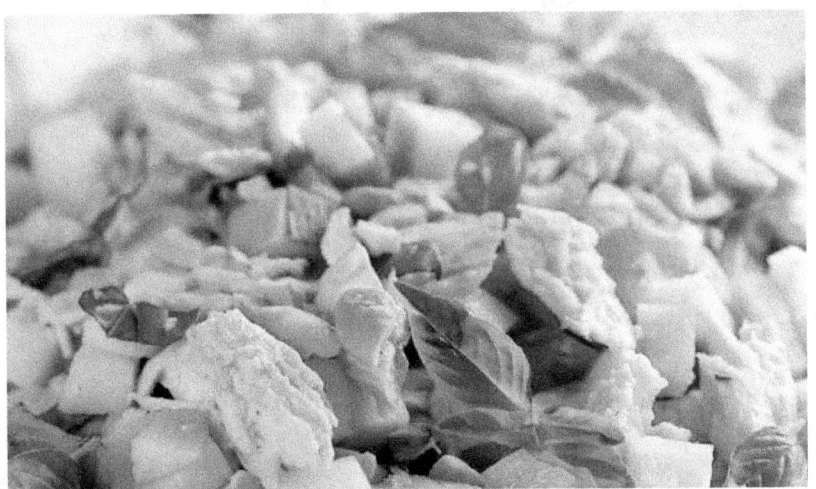

Ingredients:

- 4 oz chicken breasts, skinless and boneless, cooked
- 3 tbsp lemon juice
- 3 celery stalk, diced
- 1/8 tsp cinnamon
- 1 medium apple, cored and diced
- 2 tbsp walnuts, chopped
- Stevia to taste

Directions:

1. Cut cooked chicken into the bite size pieces.

2. Add all ingredients into the bowl and toss well until combined.
3. Place bowl in refrigerator for 20 minutes.
4. Serve chilled and enjoy.

Nutritional Value (Amount per Serving):
- Calories 448
- Fat 18.5 g
- Carbohydrates 37.1 g
- Sugar 25 g
- Protein 37.9 g
- Cholesterol 101 mg

43-Creamy Coconut Cauliflower Spinach Soup

Total Time: 45 minutes

Serves: 5 Servings

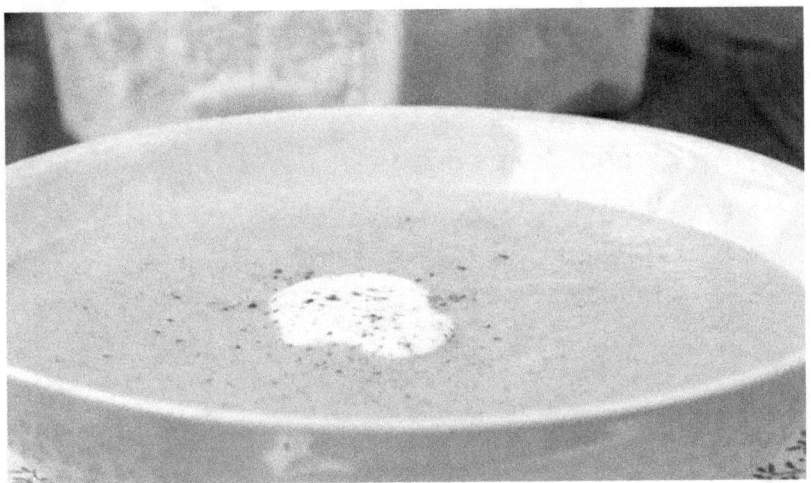

Ingredients:
- 1 lb cauliflower, chopped
- 5 watercress, chopped
- 8 cups vegetable broth
- 1/2 cup coconut milk
- 5 oz fresh spinach, chopped
- Salt

Directions:
1. Add chicken broth and cauliflower in large saucepan and bring to boil over medium heat for 15 minutes.

2. Add spinach and watercress and cook for another 10 minutes.
3. Remove from heat and using blender, puree the soup until smooth.
4. Add coconut milk and stir well.
5. Season with salt.
6. Serve hot and enjoy.

Nutritional Value (Amount per Serving):
- Calories 149
- Fat 8.2 g
- Carbohydrates 8.7 g
- Sugar 4.2 g
- Protein 11.3 g
- Cholesterol 0 mg

44-Simple Asparagus Zucchini Soup

Total Time: 40 minutes

Serves: 4 Servings

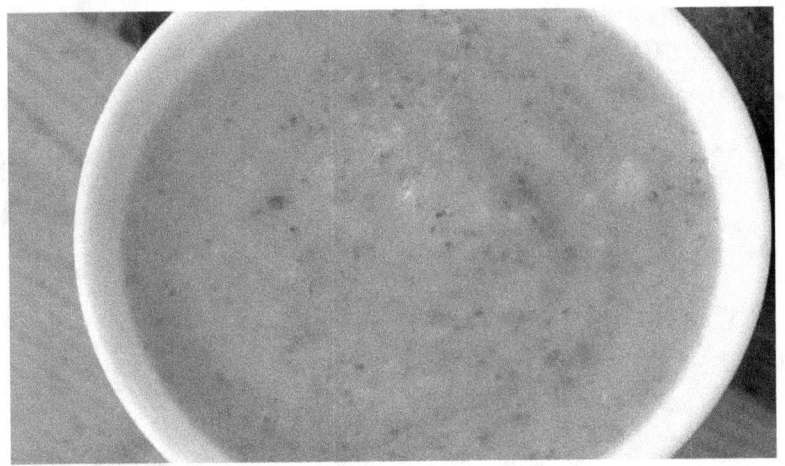

Ingredients:
- 1 lb zucchini, chopped
- 1 lb asparagus, trimmed and chopped
- 4 cups Vegetable broth
- Salt

Directions:
1. Add zucchini, asparagus, and broth in saucepan and bring to boil over medium heat for 20 minutes.
2. Remove soup from heat.
3. Using blender, puree the soup until smooth.
4. Season with salt.

5. Serve and enjoy.

Nutritional Value (Amount per Serving):
- Calories 79
- Fat 1.7 g
- Carbohydrates 9.1 g
- Sugar 4.8 g
- Protein 8.7 g
- Cholesterol 0 mg

45-Creamy Coconut Onion Soup

Total Time: 45 minutes

Serves: 4 Servings

Ingredients:
- 1 onion, sliced
- 1 leek, sliced
- 1 1/2 tbsp olive oil
- 4 cups vegetable stock
- 1 garlic clove, chopped
- 1 shallot, sliced
- Salt

Directions:
1. Add vegetable stock and olive oil in saucepan and bring to boil.
2. Add remaining ingredients and stir well.
3. Cover pan and simmer for 25 minutes.

4. Using blender, puree the soup until smooth.
5. Serve hot and enjoy.

Nutritional Value (Amount per Serving):
- Calories 90
- Fat 7.4 g
- Carbohydrates 10.1 g
- Sugar 4.1 g
- Protein 1 g
- Cholesterol 0 mg

www.ingramcontent.com/pod-product-compliance
Lightning Source LLC
Chambersburg PA
CBHW062048280526
45788CB00003B/1146